JOURNAL YOUR JOURNEY

A Self-Help Journal Guide

Jalinia Logan, LCSW-CCATP

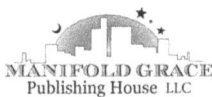

MANIFOLD GRACE
Publishing House LLC

Journal Your Journey: A Self-Help Journal Guide
Copyright, © 2022 Jalinia Logan LCSW-CCATP

ISBN: 978.1.952926.33.4

Published by Manifold Grace Publishing House, LLC
Southfield, Michigan 48033
www.manifoldgracepublishinghouse.com

Introduction

This journal was created as an additional, supportive tool to help people who are currently working towards improvement of their mental health. Using this journal does not replace therapy or receiving any other mental health services. It is simply a resource guide that helps supplement your current mental health treatment to help manage and maintain continuity of care with one's mental health outside of therapy. The journal can be utilized before and after counseling therapy. There will be prompts provided to help with guidance in journaling.

Have you ever had a journal but didn't know what to write? If so, this journal may be for you. It will help guide you as you write the narrative to discuss your inner most thoughts and feelings. This will also be a guide to help you process things for personal self-reflection.

What is one of your deepest, darkest secrets that you have, or have not, shared with someone?

What does your first healthy thought tell you to do or write? Whatever this may be, you must act on it quickly. Research says that whatever you really want to do to become better, you MUST do within 5 seconds. Otherwise, chances are you won't do it. If you go beyond the five seconds, you may start to doubt yourself, become less motivated, or even forget about it. Write out your first healthy thought below.

Page 3

Daily Thoughts

Write at least 2 words **minimum** per day for 7 days to describe how you feel.

MONDAY

Tuesday – Daily Thoughts

Two words minimum to begin to describe your thoughts or express how you are feeling.

Wednesday - Daily Thoughts

Two word minimum to begin describing your thoughts or express how you are feeling.

Thursday - Daily Thoughts

Two words minimum to begin to describe your thoughts or express how you are feeling.

Friday - Daily Thoughts

Two word minimum to begin to describe your thoughts or express how you are feeling.

Saturday - Daily Thoughts

Two words minimum to begin to describe your thoughts or express how you are feeling.

Sunday - Daily Thoughts

Two word minimum to begin to describing your thoughts or express how you are feeling.

_____

_____

_____

_____

_____

_____

_____

_____

_____

_____

_____

_____

_____

Toward the end of the week, please reflect on the words you wrote for each day. What patterns do you notice about the words you used to describe yourself or your mood each day?

What caused it?
Who caused it?
What time or part of the day did you notice the thoughts you described?

ANY ACCOMPLISHMENTS or tasks achieved, big or small. (Recognition of a completed task leads to accomplishing other tasks)

For example: making your bed
winning an award
helping someone else

Page 12

Write something kind about yourself...
True Affirmation

Think about where you are in life currently...

Now think about where you would like to be in your life.

      What would you be doing?

      Where would you be?

      What would you look like?

      What would you be wearing?

      What environments do you see yourself in?

Answering these questions should give you some idea of who you would like to become. Now focus on becoming that person **ONLY** and allow yourself to live.

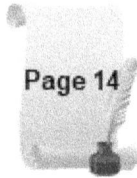

GRATITUDE NOTE

Please use this part of the journal to express some of the things you are grateful/thankful for yourself.

For example: health, family, shelter, food, water, career, helping people, small task you accomplished

Remember to acknowledge any personal accomplishments whether big or small. Small accomplishments can lead to bigger ones, so celebrate yourself and your progress because you made it! Lastly, this journal guide does not have to be the end of your thinking and writing. It is just a tool to help guide you further along in your personal journey.

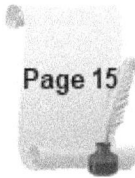

Final Excerpt

I thank GOD for giving me the strength to create this project. He only knows that it's just the beginning. I want to thank all my family and friends for your support and well wishes.

Now, I would like to thank everyone who decides to use this journal and be open about expressing some of your inner thoughts. My goal and prayer is that this tool will bless and help you in some way. Creating this journal gave me joy and I hope it inspires or motivates someone to go after their dreams. Remember, you've got this, don't rush the process - trust the process, and believe in yourself without doubt. Be true to yourself first!

Jalinia Logan, MSW, LCSW-CCATP, LPN

About the Author

Jalinia Logan is a Licensed Clinical Social Worker with a specialty as a Certified Clinical Anxiety Treatment Professional (CCATP) and a Licensed Practical Nurse. She obtained her Master's in Social Work from Chicago State University. As a health care provider, Jalinia believes in treating the whole person including biopsychosocial, physical, and spiritual. She works to help people improve towards mental and physical health. Because she has worked as a Licensed Nurse and Psychotherapist, she is able to assist people with making the connection between mental health impacts on physical health and well-being. Jalinia has worked as a nurse for 12+ years in long-term care, subacute rehab, school nursing, and as a pediatric home health nurse provider. She then went on to become a medical social worker in dialysis and hospice, a case manager at Rush University Hospital, a therapist for a group therapy practice, and now she is the founder and owner of Growth & Guidance Counseling, PC. She has been featured on Chicago's very own WGN news Daytime Talk Chicago. Jalinia's goal is to help create more opportunities in the healthcare industry for other clinicians and expand mental health services to people in need who are seeking resources/support.

You may reach Jalinia for book club appearances, speaking engagements or discussions via email: journalyourjourneynow@gmail.com

www.ingramcontent.com/pod-product-compliance
Lightning Source LLC
Chambersburg PA
CBHW052026030426
42335CB00026B/3304